Longevity Training-Book 10-Implementing the 10 Principles

This book is a transcription and reproduction of the training course materials from Course #10 "Implementing the 10 Principles"

This is the final course of the Personal Longevity Coaching Program. It is all about review of the previous courses and how to implement the 10 principles in your lives.

My goal as the developer of this training program is to help you learn the actual techniques and lifestyle to help you live decades longer. (Which I really believe is possible.)

This course also includes a couple of planning spreadsheets which are explained. Just snapshots are included in the book although you can obtain the actual spreadsheets by emailing me.

Longevity Training-Book 10-Implementing the 10 Principles

Longevity Training-Book 10-Implementing the 10 Principles

Copyright Page

The book is copyrighted for 2018

Longevity Training-Book 10-Implementing the 10 Principles

By Martin K. Ettington

ISBN: 9781792161834

Longevity Training-Book 10-Implementing the 10 Principles

Longevity Training-Book 10-Implementing the 10 Principles

Other books by Martin K. Ettington

Spiritual and Metaphysics Books:
Prophecy: A History and How to Guide
God Like Powers and Abilities
Enlightenment for Newbies
Removing Illusions to Find True
    Happiness
Using the Scientific Method to Study
    the Paranormal
A Compendium of Metaphysics and
    How to Guides (Six books
    together in one volume)
Love from the Heart
The Enlightenment Experience
Learn Your Soul's Purpose
Pursuing Enlightenment
A Modern Man's Search for Truth
Use Intuition and Prophecy to Improve
    Your Life
The Handbook of Spiritual and Energy
    Healing

Longevity & Immortality:
Physical Immortality: A History and
    How to Guide
The Commentaries of Living Immortals
Records of Extremely Long Lived
    Persons
Enlightenment and Immortality
Longevity Improvements from Science
The 10 Principles of Personal
    Longevity
Telomeres & Longevity
The Diets and Lifestyles of the Worlds
    Oldest Peoples
The Longevity Six Books Bundle

Science Fiction:
Out of This Universe
Personal Freedom-Parts 1 & 2
The Psychic Soldier Series:
    Book 1-Himalayan Journey
    Book 2-A Soldier is Born
    Book 3-Fighting For Right
    Book 4-Earth Protector
The Immortality Sci Fi Bundle

The God Like Powers Series:
Human Invisibility
Invulnerability and Shielding
Teleportation
Psychokinesis
Our Energy Body, Auras, and
Thoughtforms

The God Like Powers Series—
    Volume 1 Compilation
The Yoga Discovery Series:
Yoga-An Ancient Art Form
Hatha Yoga-Helping you Live Better
Raja Yoga-Through the Ages
The Yoga Discovery Package

Business & Coaching Books:
Creating, Paublishing, & Marketing
    Practitioner Ebooks
Building a Successful Longevity
    Coaching Business
Why Become a Coach?
The Professional Coaching Success
Trilogy
2020-Make Money Writing and Selling
    Books
The 2020 Handbook of High Paying
    Work Without a College Degree

Science, Technology, and Misc.
Future Predictions By and Engineer &
    Seer
The Unusual Science & Technology
    Bundle
The Real Atlantis-In the Eye of the
    Sahara
Are Cryptozoological Animals Real or
    Imaginary?
Real Time Travel Stories From a
    Psychic Engineer
Removing Limits On Our
    Consciousness-And
    Thinking Outside the Box
33 Incredible True Survival Stories
How to Survive Anything: From the
    Wilderness to Man Made
    Disasters
All About Mars Journeys and
    Settlement
Mining the Asteroid Belt

Ancient History
The Real Atlantis-In the Eye of the
Sahara
Ancient & Prehistoric Civilizations
Ancient & Prehistoric Civilizations-Book
    Two
The History of Antediluvian Giants
The Antediluvian History of Earth
Ancient Underground Cities and
    Tunnels
Strange Objects Which Should Not Exist

Longevity Training-Book 10-Implementing the 10 Principles

Strange and Ancient Places in the USA
A Theory of Ancient Prehistory And
        Giant Aliens
<u>Aliens and Space</u>
Aliens and Secret Technology
Aliens Are Already Among Us
Designing and Building Space Colonies
Humanity and the Universe

All About Moon Bases
All About Mars Journeys and Settlement
The Space and Aliens Six Books Bundle
A Theory of Ancient Prehistory and
        Giant Aliens
The Space Colonies and Space
        Structures Coloring Book
All About Asteroids

<u>The Longevity Training Series</u>

(A transcription of the online Multimedia Longevity Coaching Training Program)

The Personal Longevity Training Series-Book1-Long Lived Persons
The Personal Longevity Training Series-Book2-Your Soul's Purpose
The Personal Longevity Training Series-Book3-Enable Your Life Urge
The Personal Longevity Training Series-Book4-Your Spiritual Connection
The Personal Longevity Training Series-Book5-Having Love in Your Heart
The Personal Longevity Training Series-Book6-Energy Body Health
The Personal Longevity Training Series-Book7-The Science of Longevity
The Personal Longevity Training Series-Book8-Physical Body Health
The Personal Longevity Training Series-Book9-Avoiding Accidents
The Personal Longevity Training Series-Book10-Implementing These Principles

The Personal Longevity Training Series-Books One Thru Ten

These books are all available in digital and printed formats from my
website and on Amazon, Barnes & Noble, Apple ITunes, and many other sites

My Books Website is: http://mkettingtonbooks.com

Longevity Training-Book 10-Implementing the 10 Principles

<u>Signup for our Mailing List to get the following:</u>

1) A discount coupon for 25% discount on all books on our site

2) Occasional Notices of new books available

3) Occasional Email on other offerings of ours (Monthly)

Go to this link to sign-up:

http://personal-longevity.com/mkebooks/emailsignup/

And click this link to get the FREE 102 page Ebook titled "Secrets of Many Things"

If you have any questions about this book or other subjects please contact the Author at:

mke@mkettingtonbooks.com

Longevity Training-Book 10-Implementing the 10 Principles

Table of Contents

Longevity Training-Book 10-Implementing the 10 Principles

Longevity Training-Book 10-Implementing the 10 Principles

Introduction

Back in 2008 I became very interested in the field of Longevity and Physical Immortality. After a lot of research this led me to my first book on the subject "Physical Immortality: A History and How to Guide". This book was pretty popular and I wanted to continue learning about Longevity and what things we could do about it in our lives.

The subject continued to fascinate me to the point that I developed a Longevity Coaching program over a couple of years starting in 2011. This online training program was multimedia—consisting of videos, my writings on longevity to read, online exercises, and tests for each of ten courses. It also included a lot of additional resources for each course including extra courses on how to become a successful Longevity Coach. A student who completed the training and tests successfully would become certified as a "Longevity Coach" and authorized to teach this material to others.

I developed a set of ten principles on longevity which are as follows:

The 10 Principles of Personal Longevity are:

- The Reality of Long Lived People
- Defining Your Purpose in Life
- Enabling the Life Urge
- Your Spiritual Health
- Having Love in Your Heart
- Energy Body Health
- The Science of Longevity
- Physical Body Health
- Using your Intuition for Safety
- Implementation of these principles

What are the 10 Principles all about?

The Reality of Long Lived People

The first principle is where I provide lots of evidence of people who have lived well over the age of 120 years old to 150-180-200, and even a 256 year old man from China:

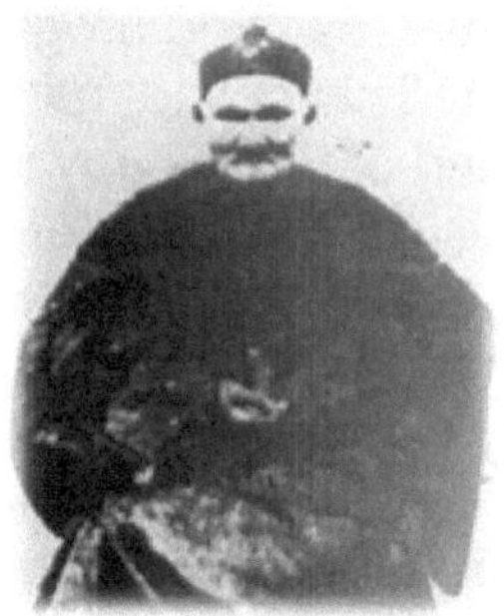

LI CHING-YUN: The Longest Lived person of record-256 Years (Source-The New York Times-May 6, 1933)

The Second Principle of Life Purpose

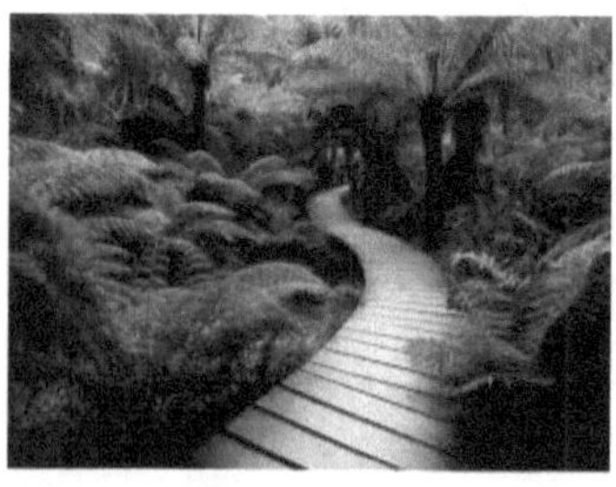

One of the things that occurred to me when I was putting the 10 principles together was that if one doesn't have a reason to live, or purpose in life--then what is the point?

This meant I had to add a very important step of how you can develop your own life purpose, or bring it up to date with your phase in life. Without reviewing your purpose-- then none of the rest of the principles matter.

Enabling the Life Urge

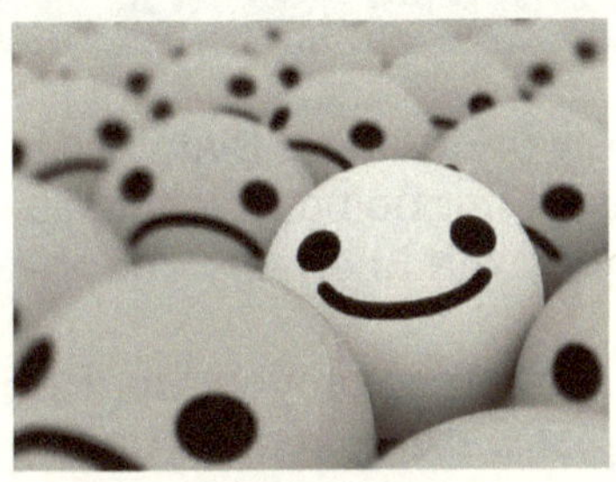

Have you ever realized how we are all programmed to expect to live through certain stages in life and then die? It's so common in our society that we don't think it odd that we expect to die at a certain age?

Have you ever heard radio ads saying "You are getting up in your sixties and seventies" so it's time to come out to our cemetery and buy a plot"

How ridiculous is this? And do you see how much our subconscious has been programmed towards death?

This principle is all about reprogramming ourselves to have a more positive outlook on life and its possibilities.

Having a Spiritual Connection in Your Life

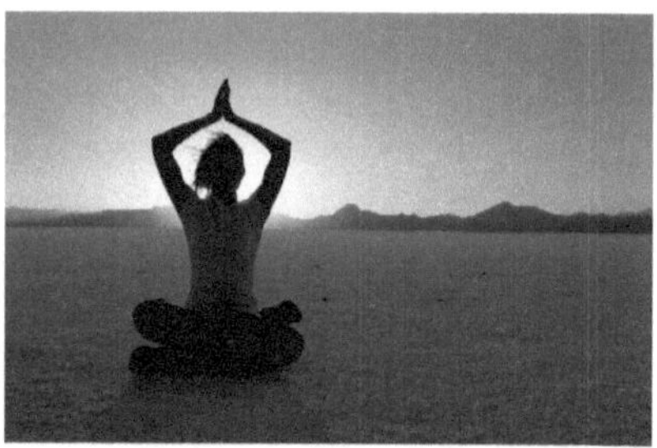

Most of us innately understand that we have a spiritual core in the center of our being. It is this spiritual core that we need to connect with to enable our physical health too.

It doesn't matter what religion you are. Regular meditation, deep prayer, or just walking in the woods helps you make and keep that connection in your life.

Having Love in Your Heart

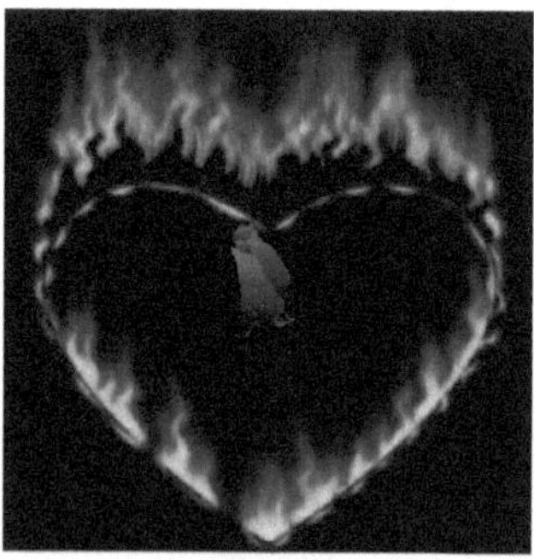

One of the most important things I learned in the last five years was that Unconditional Love is a real and physical thing. It is a powerful energy force in life and not just a philosophical belief system.

I considered it so important that I added it as a separate principle of longevity.

True Unconditional Love is healing, embodies happiness, and is a powerful part of our vital forces.

Energy Body Health

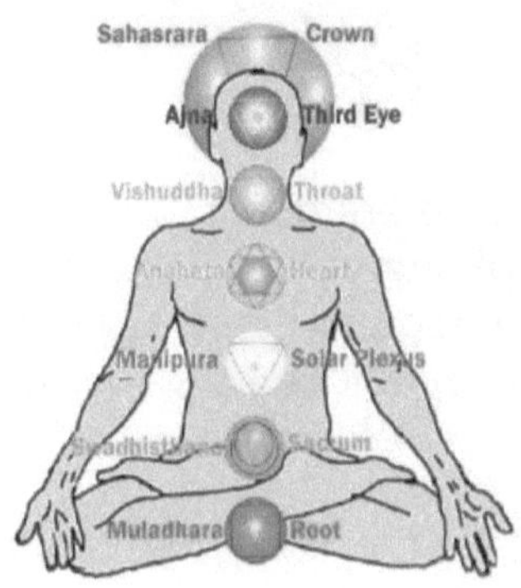

We all have an energy body which is part of our vital forces. The Indians talk about the "Chakras" and the Chinese talk about "Energy Meridians" in Acupuncture.

We should all learn different practices to keep our vital forces flowing for maximum health and vitality.

The Science of Longevity

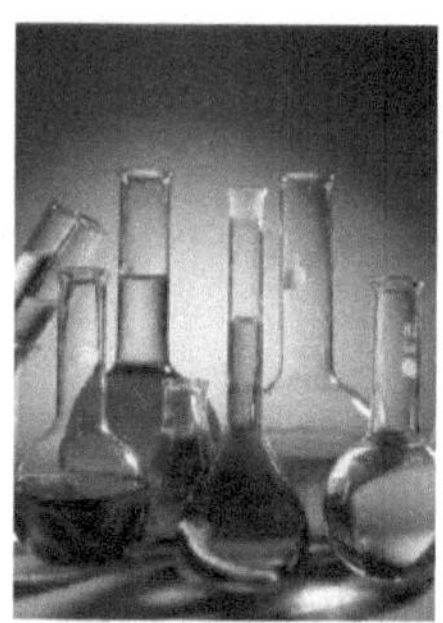

Science and Medicine are making new discoveries all the time that we can take advantage of to extend our lives. Why not take advantage of these discoveries which provide new therapies and supplements to increase our longevity.

There is also a lot we can learn from plants and animals. We all share the same genetic basis.

Some of these plants and animals live thousands of years and some cells are immortal.

What can we learn from them to apply to our lives?

Physical Body Health

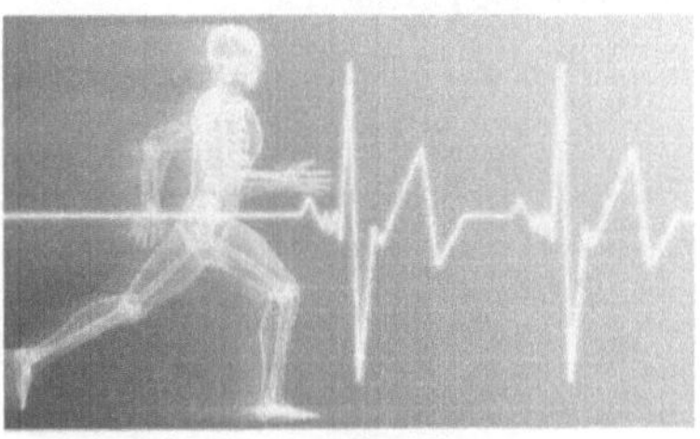

There are many types of supplements used for anti-aging for thousands of years. What can we learn about them that we can apply to our lives?

What other considerations about our physical health does nontraditional or alternative medicine offer?

Using Your Intuition for Safety

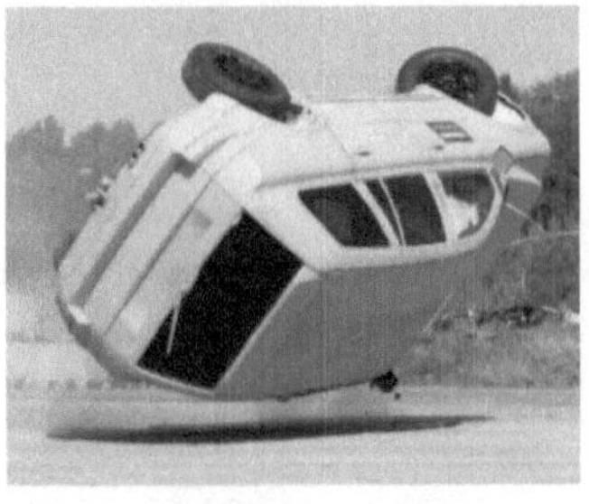

Once you have established your own long term health then what is the greatest danger you face?

ACCIDENTS

We can learn to use our intuition to make us safer as well as see potential future events which may be good too.

Longevity Training-Book 10-Implementing the 10 Principles

Why not open up to the possibilities of how our spirit has this natural ability in all of us?

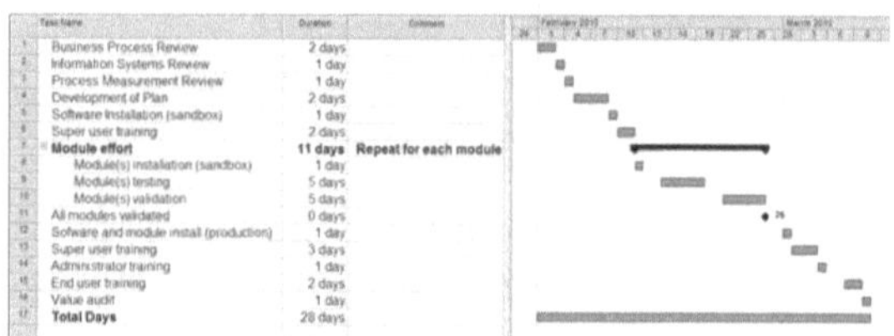

It's nice to read about all these concepts, but how can you really apply them to your own life?

This is what the chapter on implementation is all about, and it helps you plan a lifelong change in your health focus to live these principles and truly experience long term health, greater happiness, and extended longevity.

For five years I amended and improved these materials which now include a lot more information and helpful concepts for students wanting to improve their longevity and those of others.

I transcribed my videos and other materials to this book so you can read it all, and later hear it in an AudioBook.

This book is priced pretty inexpensively, compared to the online training and certification program which sells in total for $1,995 USD. If you are interested in taking the entire online program at a major discount, then please contact me at:

Marty@personal-longevity.com

Hope you enjoy these materials since when applied correctly they will significantly change your life.

PLP Concepts Overview

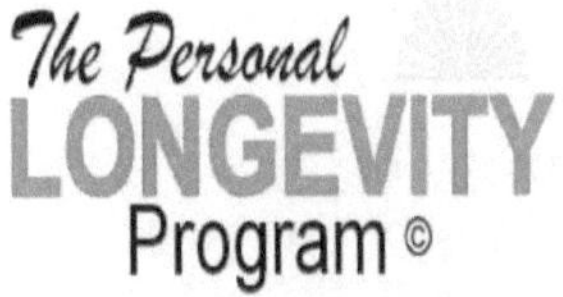

(Transcription of overview video)

Hello I'm Martin Ettington and I'd like to introduce you to the Personal Longevity Program which is an integrated holistic approach to long-term health. In this video we will only cover the high level concepts which comprise individual courses in the coaching certificate program for personal longevity.

The first concept is that long lived people exist and have existed for hundreds of thousands of years. We cover in the first course all about their records; along with people not only in places you might think like India, but in Europe and the United States-people who've lived long lives and well documented cases.

We discuss people who have lived well over the age of 120 and even the case of a Chinaman who lived to 256 years old. Plus a lot of mythology about people who have lived even longer lives so you get an idea that extending your life much longer than we think is currently medically and scientifically possible is certainly something that can happen.

The second course's concept has to do with finding your souls purpose. The point of wanting to live a long life is to know what your purpose in life is, so we go through some readings and some exercises to help you determine where soul's purpose in life is. Then doing goals as a fundamental concept so you will know the motivations in your life.

Third is the "Psychology of Living" also known by certain practitioners as "Removing the death Urge". The psychology of living has to do with seeking a positive image about your ability to live a long time. We tend to be programmed from birth about the idea that we are going to go through certain stages in our life as a child, as a teenager, and as adults. It's about reprogramming your subconscious as to the possibilities of a long life.

I've also learned in my life that it is very important to be able open your heart to unconditional love. When you're able to love unconditionally it also helps increase the strength of your immune system and fight off disease. So this is an aspect of spiritual growth. The courses also cover unconditional love and energy body forces. Managing your energy body is an important component of who you are in having energy working properly in your body and is another aspect of health for the length of longevity.

There are many types of scientific and medical research which are being done today and which will contribute to human longevity in the future.

Do you know that the average lifespan in the United States in 1900 was only about 40 years? We have doubled lifespan in the last century with current technologies but things under way in terms of scientific and medical improvements will help extend your lives further.

Also in this course on longevity we will cover a lot of the concepts which are being researched by scientists today. There are suggestions for more things you can do to do to

Longevity Training-Book 10-Implementing the 10 Principles

use this science to improve your health along with physical supplements.

A unique thing that I thought about and decided to offer in these courses has to do with all my experiences in prophecy and how I was able to change outcomes on accidents that would occur to me by using simple exercises you can learn to change these outcomes. If you're in great health often the biggest thing you have to worry about are accidents.

We also provide guidelines you can follow on a daily basis and plans you can make to live healthier and happier and have a much longer life than you ever thought possible.

Thank you for listening !

Longevity Training-Book 10-Implementing the 10 Principles

Course #10 Intro Video

(Transcription of Video)

Hello this is Marty Ettington. I'd like to welcome you to course number 10. It is a summary of longevity concepts. Congratulations if you've made it this far, going through the other nine courses.

You've learned a lot of information about how to improve your health, happiness and long-term, longevity. This course is designed as a review of the other nine courses in the PLP program. You will be reviewing in each assignment the key concepts and there will be exercises for each of those as a refresher. So after you go through the reviews of the different concepts covered in the other nine courses then the last section has to do with a review of the concepts at a high level. What we call the seven believes to help life extension and some exercises you do on creating your own path to immortality and longevity.

So again I hope you enjoy this course. This is the wrap-up of the Personal Longevity program. Thank you very much.

PLP Implementation Spreadsheets

(On using the PLP implementation word template and the PLP implementation spreadsheet (snapshots of the spreadsheets are attached)

Hello there is a document and two forms provided in course number 10 for the PLP implementation process. The word document which has a section for each of the assignments that you're given. Where you fill in the information on deciding what specific practices you would like to do. For example we could use the assignment on spiritual practices where it gives some examples about things you can do like prayer in church, or meditation, or walking in the woods, and then you would fill out some ideas of specific implementation plans to help you live that principle in your life.

The other forms that we have which down near the end of the course is the implementation spreadsheets and you're going to use this after you have decided what types of specific implementations you want to do and then here what you would do is put down by month how often or what days etc that you plan to do them. So the idea is that by going through this course and by using these two planning spreadsheets you're going to have a plan and a schedule for how you want to implement the principles in your life. Then you'll use the support system we have with our webinars and other blogs and follow up too so we can help monitor you and help give you feedback on how you're doing on implementing these things. So good luck

Longevity Training-Book 10-Implementing the 10 Principles

on implementing the Personal Longevity Program in your life. Thank you.

(See a snapshot of the longevity implementation spreadsheets below)

Longevity Training-Book 10-Implementing the 10 Principles

Longevity Intial Review Questions and Scores:

Name of Client:

Interview Date:

Score of -5=Needs Work 0=Average 5=Adept or complete

The 10 Principles	Questions	Answers	Scores	Weight	Net Score	Additional Reasons for Score
Real Long lived people	Do you believe in the records of long lived persons over the age of 150 years old?			1	0	
	How long do you think a person can live?			1	0	
	How long do you want to live and why?			2	0	
Life Purpose	What is your life purpose?			2	0	
	Is your Purpose Realistic?			1	0	
Life Urge	Are you open to living a long time?			3	0	
	Are you worried about being immobile or a shutin?			1	0	
	In what ways do you believe your life is physically limited?			3	0	
Spiritual connection	Do you have a spiritual connection?			2	0	
	Do you work on your spiritual connection on a regular basis with standard practices?			3	0	
	Any unusual beliefs about your spirit or spiritual connection?			1	0	
Unconditional Love (UL)	Do you know what unconditional love is? (Define)			1	0	

G20 | fx

Name of Client:

Start Date:

Instructions--This page summarizes the activities performed for each Practice Page

Summary of Activities Each Month

TAB#	Activity Area	Specific Practice/Exercise/Regimen	Month1	Month2	Month3	Month4	Month5	Month6	Month7	Month8	Month9	Month10	Month11	Month12
P2	Your Soul's Purpose and Goals	Choice P2	comment,	comment,	0	0	0	0	0	0	0	0	0	0
P3	Affirmations for Living	Choice P3	0	0	0	0	0	0	0	0	0	0	0	0
P4	Spiritual Growth Plans	Choice P4	0	0	0	0	0	0	0	0	0	0	0	0
P5	Mastering Your Energy Body	Choice P5	0	0	0	0	0	0	0	0	0	0	0	0
P6	Supplements and Natural Health	Choice P6	0	0	0	0	0	0	0	0	0	0	0	0
P7	Learning to Avoid Accidents	Choice P7	0	0	0	0	0	0	0	0	0	0	0	0
P8	Plan for Exercising your Physical Body	Choice P8	0	0	0	0	0	0	0	0	0	0	0	0

Longevity Training-Book 10-Implementing the 10 Principles

PLP Implementation Planning Instructions

Assignment--Long Lived People:

The information about long lived people is mainly to convince the reader that people can really live to over the age of 150 years. You become more readily aware of these people through studying the specifics of their lives and what they did to maintain health and longevity so you can now apply many of the techniques you have learned into everyday practice in your life.

Do you have any doubts at this point that these people really lived this long? What are these doubts?

If so, what additional research can you do to convince yourself of the reality of these long lived people?

What are three practices you can take forward with you that were commonly practiced amongst long lived people that you have researched from course 2? Write these three practices down. Make sure to be specific, measurable, attainable, relevant and trackable!

1.

2.

3.

Longevity Training-Book 10-Implementing the 10 Principles

Assignment: Soul Purpose:

Do you have a written Soul Purpose statement? What is it?-keeping it in 2-4 sentences?

Example of a Soul Purpose Statement:

"My purpose in life is to help people develop a holistic philosophy in their lives for long term health, greater happiness and extended longevity" –By Martin K. Ettington

There are many resources for developing and updating your Soul's Purpose.

This link is for Soul Purpose videos on YouTube

Have you thought about your goals resulting from this statement? Write them down. Make sure to be specific, measurable, attainable, relevant, and trackable!

Do you see yourself realistically living up to your Soul Purpose Statement?

If so, visualize the way you look, think and feel for ten or more minutes in a meditative state of being calm and grounded in your thoughts and actions.

If not, what are your plans to either do this yourself with the exercises in Course #2 or to find a Life Purpose Coach to help you with this process?

Assignment: The Psychology of Living

Do you have a plan for building your positive affirmations? If so, write them down below.

If you would like additional information on positive affirmations check out the following below:

- Louise Hay, founder of Hay House Publishing, has many books and CDs on affirmations for various areas in your life including health, relationships and career.

- THE PRESENT MOMENT: 365 DAILY AFFIRMATIONS BY LOUISE HAY

If not, what could you do in terms of recordings, meetings you attend, videos you watch, or just discussions with friends to build your life urge and remove the death urge?

Please write down what you can do to change your daily psychology to a psychology of living, as you previously studied about earlier.

Make a list of your favorite affirmations and write them down on cards to keep with you in your pocket or hand out to others.

Longevity Training-Book 10-Implementing the 10 Principles

Assignment: Spiritual Practices

Write down what spiritual practices you do now, and which ones you would like to add on a regular basis to help life extension. Again, there are lots of options--the key is to do one regularly.

Examples of Spiritual Practices:

- Prayer in Church
- Meditation—various forms
- Walking in the woods and communing with Nature

Also note why you think these new spiritual practices will help your life extension.

Create an affirmation that you can take with you when you work on your spiritual practices. Write it down on a card that you can have available to you

Example:

-"I have practiced chi-gong for 18 years and it really makes me feel centered and more aware of my thoughts. I just recently found out about a new practice, Falun Dafa and would like to try it to meet other spiritual people and see if I can use both of the practices in my life to further better my mind-body connection. I believe this can increase my life extension because I have found studies in my research that talk about falun dafa and its importance to your overall health and longevity with scientific facts and testimonials."

Longevity Training-Book 10-Implementing the 10 Principles

Assignment: Unconditional Love

Planning some specific practices to work on experiencing unconditional love is an important practice to better yourself along the path to your personal longevity, health and happiness.

This can be exercises like the heart rose exercise--many types on YouTube, or can be the DeMartini method--which you can take classes on.

Here is a link to books you can also buy on unconditional love:

Unconditional Love Books

Write down the practices have you chosen to practice on a regular basis to experience unconditional love and what your reasoning is for choosing them

Assignment: The Energy Body

Write down what vital forces practices you do presently, and which ones you plan to start to energize your body. This is something that you should practice at least weekly and there are many types of instructors to choose from.

Examples:

- Counseling
- Reiki Healing
- Aura Cleansings
- Acupressure
- Acupuncture
- Spiritual Projection
- Chi Gong
- etc.

Why have you chosen this practice and what effects do you expect it to have on you?

A diary can be a great way of keeping track of your progress on your energy body, noting how you feel after each and every practice. This will give you an idea a year from now on which ones are more effective for you and your lifestyle.

Longevity Training-Book 10-Implementing the 10 Principles

Assignment: Your Physical Body

This is a good place to write down all of the things you are doing to take care of your physical body such as:

- Exercises
- Diet
- Cleanliness

What other techniques have you learned from reading up on current scientific and medical thought to apply to your overall health?

- Resveratrol Supplements
- Ginseng Supplements

Please also write down what herbal supplements or other natural food and herbal remedies you might want to start taking. (This is not required and is totally up to your discretion and your doctor's advice)

Or you can all check these online resources:

- The Complete Book of Herbs: A Practical Guide to Growing and Using Herbs
- http://www.altnature.com/bookstore.htm
- The Herb Book by John Lust
- The Pill Book Guide to Natural Medicines Michael Murray N.D.
- Use and Abuse of Herbs Karen Vaughn

Assignment: Avoiding Accidents

A big part of learning to use your intuition to enjoy greater personal safety is to exercise your abilities to see future potential paths in your life.

Fortune telling exercises help with this a lot.

In the prophecy book, you will find that chapter 6 lists over 100 types of fortune telling in detail. Some examples of the ones discussed at length include:

- The IChing
- Crystal Balls
- Tarot Cards

Choose a practice you are comfortable with and set a schedule to practice it on a regular basis to develop your skills to see future events.

Longevity Training-Book 10-Implementing the 10 Principles

Assignment: Your Own Path

In this exercise you will work on customizing your usage of the principles you learned in this entire certificate program:

Write down the six goals for life extension from chapter 15 of "Physical Immortality: A History and How to Guide" and write down why you think each of these goals are important for long term health and longevity

Download the spreadsheet below titled "plp-lifestyle planning". Then fill out this sheet about what specific actions you will take for the different topics in the left column to improve your health, happiness, and length of living.

You should fill in details of your plans for each month for the first year. You are encouraged to keep using this planning sheet for subsequent years as well!

Finances for Long Lived People

Introduction-Finances of Long Lived People

My focus for years now has been how to help people optimize their long term health and improve their overall Longevity.

My training programs teach about how to integrate Spirit, Mind, and Body as part of that optimization process. We also teach important principles which also affect longevity such as "Life Purpose" and using Intuition for Safety.

However, one area I've pretty much neglected is what to do about your long term finances.

The problem is that the planning horizon for individuals and governments is now much shorter than an individual's potential longevity.

So what will happen if you live a long time? Will you run out of money and become homeless? Or dependent on family and government to live instead of maintaining your independence?

The purpose of this book is to address these issues and help you develop really long term financial plans which will withstand the uncertainties of time

Within our Longevity Research we found out, that if one doesn't have a reason to live, or have a purpose in life—then what is the point?

This means a very important step to developing longevity is how you can develop your own positive life purpose, or bring it up to date with your phase in life. Without reviewing your purpose—none of the rest of the longevity principles matter.

****

I'm not going to get into all of the principles in detail here--since that is part of the Longevity Coaching training, but I wanted to give you the reader just a little flavor of what this subject is all about.

Current Financial Planning Strategies

Today, when people plan for their retirement and their finances for later in life they usually look at a retirement from the late fifties to the eighties.

This is a natural assumption, since most people believe that they will only live into their eighties at the most. Why bother planning for a much longer life?--since it's pretty unlikely anyway.

Most of these plans revolve around having the following financial assets:

- Personal Savings
- Pensions
- Social Security & Medicare

The problem is that personal savings are not allocated for an individual to last beyond their eighties, Pensions are underfunded, and government support obligations are much greater than the government can cover in the long run.

Therefore, personal savings will eventually run out, and government support and/or pensions will be eventually be cut way back.

With these types of retirement planning assumptions you are almost guaranteed to become indigent if you live into your nineties or beyond.

The Uncertainties of Planning for the Future

In addition, we like to think that our society is stable, that existing financial investments will always work, and that it is possible to plan for our financial futures.

The problem with this thinking is that over 100 years or more, societies and the structure of civilization changes dramatically--and so do investment and work opportunities.

Let's look at some examples of how the world has changed in the last 100 years in ways which affect investments, careers, and other opportunities:

1) 100 years ago in 1914, the world was at the beginning of World War 1 and the political structure of the world was about to have major re-alignments. The governments and legal boundaries of much of the world changed in the next few years.

2) Communism in Russia was adopted in 1917 which totally changed the idea of the validity of business and owning property.

3) WW2 further changed the power alignment of the world, and therefore how people could invest and where they could invest.

4) The Computer revolution started in the late 1940s and is still going. Entire industries have grown up (or died) based on the growth of computer technology or the Internet.

5) Most of the top companies in the United States 100 years ago are gone today with only a few exceptions, while the top companies in the US didn't exist 20 years ago. So

professions and job opportunities have changed dramatically.

6) The Great Depression in the 1930s and more recently the Great Recession in 2008 changed the world economy, opportunities, and investments.

What can we learn from past events:

1) Job and Economic opportunities change over time
2) Investments in one era may not be successful in another era.
3) Breakdowns of civilization occur pretty frequently on the scale of 100 years.

Longevity Training-Book 10-Implementing the 10 Principles

A Really Long Term Financial Strategy

Okay--so with the preceding knowledge and assumptions, we need to come up with a completely different plan to support your life if you are going to live to 100 years or significantly more.

This means setting some new guidelines about what you will need to survive in the long term:

1) We will assume that you need to have continually renewing sources of investment to provide long term income.

2) That government or corporate pensions may be cut back significantly or go away completely.

3) That work can be done at any age, as long as you have your "mind" and work of some type is good for your health.

4) Your experience with previous work and in life has become more and more important as the knowledge economy grows.

These new guidelines will allow you to make more realistic plans to help build your financial future

What Type of Work can you do?

You should get used to the idea that if you choose to do so, you can be in the workforce for your entire life--instead of having to retire at some point.

This is due to several factors:

1) With the aging of the Baby Boomer generation and many of them retiring, there are many more opportunities for skilled old workers now and in the future.

2) The fact of the worldwide internet and many types of work that can be done from home removes a barrier to many persons who would like to stay home to work.

3) Starting your own business is possible at any age, and is a great option for older workers.

Let's go into these three factors in more detail:

Baby Boomers Retiring:

Baby Boomers retiring from the workforce will create up to 50,000,000 new jobs in the United States by 2020. That is a lot of jobs and professions which need to be filled.

If you have the right experience and skills--even if you are older--you can take advantage of this demographic bomb.

Work at Home

According to work at home Census numbers from 2010, the percentage of people working at home rose to 4.3% of the working age population.

This percentage of the population is going up every year, so if you want to work at home, now is a good time.

Being older, you may not want to travel much or have to commute to an office every day. These days, working at home has become very feasible and the number of opportunities is growing daily.

Starting your own business

Starting your own new business is a great idea at any age. Especially since when you reach your 50s most companies will not want to hire you anyway due to your age.

However, if you are the owner of the company--you make the rules!

Having your own business is a lot of work--but can also be extremely gratifying, and be the implementation of your passions and your life's mission.

Longevity Training-Book 10-Implementing the 10 Principles

What are the best Long Term Investments?

All investments are cyclical, and no investment can be said to be the "Best for the Long Term".

What a really smart long term investor needs to do is to plan a diversification strategy so that not all their eggs are held in one basket.

Given that investments are all moving in long term cycles, you want to be positioned to be broadly balanced--no matter how the economy is where you live.
Major types of investments include but aren't limited to:

- Real Estate
- Commodities
- Stocks
- Bonds

You should plan to hold positions in all of these areas, but re-balance them at least yearly based on economic outlooks.

This will give you the most investment security in the long run--but be aware, in the really long run governments are overthrown, financial assumptions changes, private property is nationalized--so don't become totally dependent on static investments.

Building your Long Range Financial Plan

Now that we have taken a new look at assumptions about long term finances, we can finally turn to developing our own long term financial plan.

1) The first part of your plan should be what type of work you want to do?

My belief is that the coming changes in our society and cyclical economic cycles have a good chance of wiping out any investments you have. These cycles easily happen in 100 year timeframes and less--so the only security you have is really in what you know and what you can do. There is no reason that a healthy person in their sixties and older can't start a new career.

So work on finding something you can be passionate about, get what additional training you need, and launch your new career.

Participating in the workforce is really the only security any of us will have in the long term.

2) Investments

Plan a diversity of investments to cover all of the main investment areas--Real Estate, commodities, stocks, and bonds--and anything else you can think of.

Make sure to spread your risk and re-balance your portfolio at least yearly depending on economic and market conditions.

Longevity Training-Book 10-Implementing the 10 Principles

Summary-Finances of Long Lived People

In this short EBook we took at a look at conventional assumptions about financial planning to show that many current assumptions for the very long term are bad assumptions.

The knowledgeable person who is planning to live an active life decades beyond the normal lifespan needs to think outside of the box to come up with other options.

Ultimately, the only security any of us have in how we live in society is in what we know and the skills we have.
As long as we have our long term health, and long term planning for financial security, we can be assured of living through any tough times to come--and thriving in the process.

Summary

I started my research on Longevity in 2009 and developed the Personal Longevity multi-media coaching program starting in 2011.

I feel strongly that we all can learn the processes and techniques to learn to live decades longer than society thinks we can.

By taking care of your body, your mind, and connecting to the universal spirit you can dramatically change your life.

I hope the teachings of this longevity training series will be something you will practice and will benefit you greatly in the future.

Best Wishes to you all!

Martin K. Ettington

Email: marty@personal-longevity.com

www.ingramcontent.com/pod-product-compliance
Lightning Source LLC
Chambersburg PA
CBHW051235250726
48655CB00006B/2776